Destination From Infertility to Children:
A Love Story

J.R. Glenn

Published by J.R. Glenn

To my wife and children. Life takes us down some great paths and certain people cross our paths that leave us ever changed from their impressions upon our lives. Thank you for leaving your great impressions upon my life.

It was August 2005 and I met this woman that I was drawn to like no other woman. I was dating many women and enjoying the single life when Tracey came along and grabbed my attention. I wasn't expecting her to show up. I had never talked to her before. I had seen her at various places such as stores and school events.

However, I didn't really talk to

her because I was dating other

women and she was married at

first and later was dating other

men after her divorce. Our paths

hadn't crossed again since she

had become divorced.

One day our paths crossed

where she and I had our first

interaction with one another. We joked lightly with one another and kidded, picked at each other like a brother and sister would do or like great friends would do. The only problem was this was our first interaction with each other. Talk about mannerisms and all of the formal things that come along with meeting someone that you find attractive

We instantly felt that push and pull force of interest in each other and wanted to explore that more. This woman was different than the ones I had been dating. She was feisty and always had something to flirt with me right back. As the weeks turned into months and the months turned into a year, we decided to get married the next August.

Getting married was a passing thought before I met her but, after she and I met I noticed how a longing to be married to her kept lingering deep in my soul. It was weird, as I have never experienced that feeling before. I was used to dating many women and just enjoying life with whatever new adventure would come my way.

We were married for a year, getting to know one another. I mean really know one another. I found out fast that I had to keep my bathroom a certain way and that she didn't mind cooking; however, I best be there when she was cooking. She would get upset if I wasn't around when she cooked. I also, found out really fast that she didn't approve of my computer desk being located in the dining room/kitchen area. It needed to leave that area according to my new wife. Wow, this hadn't been a problem before now. So, what is the big deal I thought. Later, I decided to challenge her on that subject. Boy, was I wrong to do that, she stated that she didn't want that eye sore in the kitchen/dining area. With much persuasion, I moved the computer desk to the basement where it would be out of sight and out of mind. That first year of marriage was an adjustment for both of us. We both were learning how to live with another person since I had never done that before and it had been a couple years since she was married and had done that. It is a huge adjustment when you are married to another human being that you care for but that doesn't think like you do. You find out fast how your differences can affect one another along with the adjustment of building your new life together with the person you see day in and day out. You go to bed and the person is there. The next morning you wake up and they are there. This was a nice adjustment but, it still took time.

My new wife had children from her first marriage and she

had her tubes tied as she

stated, "I didn't want any more

children with that man I was

married to." She said, "He didn't

help me raise the children and I

didn't love him enough to have

anymore." Fair enough I thought

to myself. I understood where

she was coming from. I couldn't

blame her for not wanting

anymore children with her first

husband either. I couldn't and still can't stand him. I know that is not very nice since we are to love our neighbor. I do my neighbor, just stay over there though out of sight.

At first, I didn't care for any children of my own. I didn't really have the desire to have children in the beginning however, as time would pass by I began to have this desire that was unshakeable deep in my soul. It was gut wrenching, with a desire to have a child with my wife whose tubes were tied. I thought to myself, while trying to extinguish that fire, there was no way mortally possible that she could have a child with me in her current state of her tubes being tied. Do you know what the odds are of conceiving with your tubes tied? That is 99.9 percent chance of not happening. By the way, my wife was very fertile. She told me that she conceived through a Deppro shot and through her other birth control medicines. She said the tubal was the only thing that worked for her. I didn't' care at the time one way

or another. But, like I said earlier

a deep heartfelt yearning

swelled up deep within my soul

to have children with my wife

who was practically infertile

now. By our second year in

marriage, we were exploring the

different possibilities to get her

tubal reversal in order to have

children. That was an

experience that was up hill in every stance. We didn't know where to go, who to talk to, nor what to do. I wish there was counselling out there for couples struggling with infertility. We chose a doctor who was nationally acclaimed at having a successful tubal reversal program. Recovery would take a couple weeks and they stated that would be best route for us.

Well, $6,000 later tubal reversal
was completed. That whole
process was an emotional wreck
for both my wife and me. I was
devastated that she had to have
surgery for them to reverse her
tubal reversal. She has lost
sensation feeling in that area as
a side effect. The doctor stated
that she had 5.5 cm of the

normal 8 cm left of fallopian tube left to conceive with. I asked, "Was that good?" The doctor stated, "That is about average after a tubal reversal." So, they sent us on our way and called the day after surgery to see how Tracey was doing. I stated that she was in pain but up and walking some. She doesn't remember any of that to this day because of the high-powered pain medicine they had given her to dial back the pain. We headed home and I noticed there was some sort of loss of communication that we had. It wasn't a whole lot but may a misunderstanding that needed to be sorted out. She and I struggled with communication about our true feelings. I guess it was that we didn't want to hurt the other persons feelings.

We tried to have children for a year and a half after the tubal reversal surgery with no success. We both were frustrated and questioned everything. This was the beginning of the darkness that we were about to embark upon.

Tracey decided to go back to school with my support and encouragement in order to help her advance within the company she worked for. This was probably at first sight an accident waiting to happen. Who knew the Christian college she went to would offer free counseling sessions for couples like us who had so many miscommunication skillsets and infertility problems along with now financial difficulties. We both opened Facebook social media and began talking to previous people from previous relationships and various friends. We were seeking whatever attention that we could get from anyone that would hear us out. It was like we were strangers living together with

different dreams and ambitions.

We walked on eggshells with

each other during this time. We

didn't talk except to mistreat

each other with words.

Infertility was defeating us.

We had begun down the

destructive path of hurting one

another's feelings and not

displaying empathy to one another. We were not talking because of the hurt and pain associated with infertility and our communication dysfunction. We didn't know at the time why we couldn't stand to be in the same room with each other but, looking back we both know that miscommunication and misunderstanding about the infertility and each other's desires was the culprit.

We decided to go to the local hospital along with talking with our local doctor to find out other options on our own about infertility treatment. We were told about invitro-fertilization. Wow, what a huge daunting word, invitro-fertilization. Isn't that what they do to sheep or cows? Surely not on humans or my wife. I knew she may have been difficult to live with, as was I; but, I didn't want her hurt from some experimentation. Also, the thought of playing God with the medical advances that were available weighed heavy on us. However, that drive and yearning to have children was still deeply embedded within our soul. Evidently, both of us felt strongly for having children with each other because my wife, Tracey, was a trooper in the fact of not telling me, "NO, I will not have children with you, find someone else." She stated that she was done having children with her last husband and anyone else who had asked her to have children. She never

once told me those words.

Instead, it was let's check into it

and learn more. We both

became frustrated with the

process and the barriers that we

were up against. We lost

communication in the process.

Her ex-husband was in the

background manipulating

Tracey by trying to withhold the

children from seeing her and not willing to buy them any clothes or school supplies. They left the financial burden on us along with trying to keep the children away by dictating the times she could pick them up. For example, she would pick them up always from their dad's house at 6pm after work. He began stating that she couldn't pick them up until 8pm or something crazy to be difficult. He never would meet in the middle and be sensible. She always had to go to his house to pick them up for he rarely if ever brought them to our home. It was crazy to say the least and not really the extra burden that we needed with our current struggles. However, evidently, we were able to make it through that and are able to write about it today, some 10 years later.

When we decided to seek help from the local hospital that would eventually help lead us down the path of invitro-fertilization. We were told that I, the male, should have been tested long before my wife had to undergo the surgery of tubal reversal. After meeting with the doctors and nurses on the invitro-fertilization team we knew that we were where we should've been to begin with. This was year 2008, and remember we began this planning and conversation after getting married in August 2006. By 2007, Tracey had her tubal reversal surgery, which didn't work for us. This was a waste of time and money for us not to mention added stress and division that was created from the lack of support and help that we needed.

When we met with the invitro-fertilization doctors they immediately recommended testing me in order for them to be able to make a plan of how to help us with our infertility treatment. This plan scared us because of the unknowns, the financial burden, and the low chances of success to achieve our dreams of having children together. We both still had the yearning to have children with each other; however, that dream was just that a dream. We had walls at every turn that we made. Talk about feeling stuck and beat down, we did. We were so much so that we began to argue and mistreat one another out of lack of communication of our needs and desires.

The process of invitro-fertilization scared us to death and we had mixed feelings since the process of the tubal reversal was so stressful and had failed for us. The staff was helpful and guided us with support and direction through the process of the invitro-fertilization. We both walked out of the doctor's visit with ease and felt like this is what we needed to do in order to achieve our dream of having children together. We still had a few questions as to how this process would look, what was the financial burden, what pain and sacrifices would we make? We found out that it was expensive and that we had a 35% chance of it working for us. The positive was that Tracey had been able to conceive and birth children in the past so that would help increase the odds. We struggled over the process and I felt as if Tracey wasn't interested in going through the process after our first meeting with the invitro-fertilization doctors because of the unknowns. This was devastating to me and I felt as if she was giving up on the dream. I felt mislead and betrayed. I still remember sitting outside a pizza place that we had chosen to eat lunch at and talking after the meeting with the doctors. She told me that she wasn't sure that she wanted to go down this path and wondered if it were best for us to just not have children. That hit me like a sword to the heart. I felt crushed, devastated, sad, and hurt at the same time and the yearning deep in my heart and soul was stronger than ever. I didn't know how to share with her my feelings so I told her, "Either you have children with me or maybe we should consider divorce." That was the ultimate blow. I saw the hurt and felt the hurt in her eyes, emotions, body language, and the tension and mistrust was established. The tension was so strong that it couldn't be cut with a knife. I was hurt and now I had hurt her all over a misunderstanding and miscommunication about this infertility problem that we had.

From this was the downward spiral of trust being broken and the arguments began between us. We decided to go through the invitro-fertilization process even with the troubles in order to achieve our dreams and hope that would correct the hurt that was brought on between us with our misunderstandings and miscommunication. It felt like we were the new Hatfield's and McCoy's with our misunderstandings and miscommunications. We found out that I was the problem that can keeping us from getting pregnant. Who knew that much of the time the problem lies within the male? They stated that I had a few healthy sperm cells but very few which lead the doctors to decide to use the assistive reproduction process or artificial insemination in a pea tree dish. This was the only way to get the sperm and egg fertilized with the problems that were in place. This was embarrassing and disheartening news to know that I was broken. I was relieved to know the doctors could help but, wow, what a blow to find out that I was the problem and that my wife had been through hell to have children with me. We were both upset and felt hurt and betrayed from the news and misguidance from the tubal reversal doctor and the misunderstanding of infertility.

In February 2008, we had begun our adventure into invitro-fertilization. We had many of our questions answered as to how the process was going to be. We found out they were going to give my wife medication to stimulate her ovaries to produce many eggs which would be extracted or harvested to be fertilized in a pea tree dish. The wonders of science and the advancement of medical technology are marvelous and scary. After the eggs were extracted, harvested, and fertilized we returned to the hospital two days later where Tracey would be impregnated with the implantation of the fertilize embryo. She had to be placed on so many medicines to trick her body into being

pregnant in order to stop or

prevent her body from expelling

the embryo and accept the

embryo. This made her a basket

of hormones to say the least.

She had to have shots in her

abdomen and buttocks daily to

stimulate and begin the process

of tricking her body into holding

on to the embryo and thinking

that she was pregnant. Nine

months later, our daughter

arrived. She was beautiful, a

blessing from heaven. Our

dream had been achieved and

the yearning deep within my

heart and soul had been

satisfied and was no longer

weighing deep in my heart.

The stress of the infertility, miscommunication, financial instability, and financial cost of the process along with the emotional stress caused from the burdens of life, her ex-husband, work, schooling, and us fighting from misunderstandings and miscommunications played heavy in our discombobulation and discontentment with one another. This process nearly caused us to divorce. We ended up turning to social media during the following months to talk to people who would listen to us since we quit listening to each other. This opened the door for infidelity and problems on top of communication problems. While my wife was in school she received an email offering

counseling to married couples

struggling as we were. She

asked her classmates if they

received an email about

counseling services and they

stated they didn't know what she

was talking about. So, this was

either divine intervention or a

hoax. She contacted the lady

back and we were scheduled to

go through counseling. This helped us to learn who we are and what we wanted out of our life and marriage. This gave us the opportunity to grow and learn how to communicate with each other better. We gained so many tools for our tool bag although we were still broken just not as badly broken. We were on the way to mending the fences. I still felt lonely on the inside and felt as if she wasn't truly interested in me. I guess she felt the same but, I didn't know for sure. We continued to go through counseling which helped us greatly. We decided to go back through the invitro-fertilization process again in which we were blessed with a handsome son. The time has passed and the communication is somewhat better; however, we still have somethings to do or work on to create the wonderful marriage that we had before all the problems that has plagued us such as: infertility, miscommunication, social media which lead to infidelity, and financial struggles that were all a part of the struggles.